Meditation

A Compilation Of Guided Meditations And Mindfulness
Exercises: Managing Your Eco-Anxiety

I0083597

*(The Straightforward Guide To Effective Daily Mindfulness
Practice)*

Demarcus Melton

TABLE OF CONTENT

Reduced Stress And Anxiety

It is essential to first comprehend what tension and anxiety are and how they impact the body. Positive or negative stress is the body's natural response to obstacles or demands. Positive stress, also known as eustress, can inspire us to attain our goals and perform at our best. In contrast, negative stress or distress can negatively impact our health and well-being.

Anxiety is a normal reaction to stress, characterized by feelings of worry, dread, and unease. When we experience anxiety, our bodies go into "fight or flight" mode, producing hormones such as adrenaline and cortisol in preparation for facing the perceived threat. Anxiety can be advantageous in small doses because it helps us to remain alert and focused. However, chronic anxiety can have detrimental effects on our health, including an increased risk of cardiovascular disease and a compromised immune system.

It has been demonstrated that meditation is an effective method for reducing tension and anxiety. It functions by calming the mind and body and fostering relaxation and inner serenity. We can program our minds to respond to stress in a more balanced and healthy manner by meditating regularly.

One of the primary mechanisms by which meditation reduces tension and anxiety is by regulating the activity of the amygdala, the brain region responsible for processing fear and anxiety. When we are agitated or anxious, the amygdala becomes overactive, resulting in an increase in stress hormone production and a heightened state of alertness.

Meditation has been shown to reduce amygdala activity, resulting in a decrease in stress hormones and a tranquil state of mind. Meditation can also increase activity in the prefrontal cortex, the region of the brain responsible for reasoning and making decisions. In stressful situations, this can enable us to think more clearly and make better decisions.

Meditation also reduces tension and anxiety by stimulating the relaxation response. The relaxation response is a condition of profound rest that opposes the "fight or flight" response triggered by stress. When the relaxation response is activated, our heart rate and respiration rate decrease, and our muscles relax. This can aid in reducing anxiety and fostering a sense of calm and well-being.

Meditation has a number of physiological benefits that can aid in tension and anxiety reduction. It has been shown to reduce blood pressure, enhance immune function, and alleviate chronic pain. These effects can aid in alleviating the physical manifestations of tension and anxiety, such as headaches and stomach aches. It can also help us develop greater self-awareness and mindfulness, allowing us to better comprehend our thoughts, emotions, and stress responses. This can allow us to respond to stress in a more healthful and balanced manner.

Overall, the benefits of meditation for tension and anxiety reduction are evident. By meditating consistently, we can train our mind and body to respond to stress in a more balanced and healthy manner, resulting in enhanced physical and mental health.

Types Of Meditation

Meditation is the umbrella term in the field of nursing for the various methods of achieving a tranquil state of mind. There are numerous varieties of meditation and relaxation techniques that incorporate meditation. Everyone's constant objective is to attain inner serenity.

Examples of meditative practices include:

The practice of guided meditation. Typically referred to as a guided basic cognitive process or mental representation, in this form of meditation you create mental images of locations or objects that you find relaxing.

You utilize as many of your senses as possible, including smells, sights, noises, and textures. A guide or instructor can help you become a junction rectifier using this method.

Mantra meditation. For the duration of this meditation technique, you silently repeat a tranquil word, thought, or phrase to prevent distracting thoughts.

The practice of mindfulness meditation. This form of meditation requires awareness or a heightened awareness, as well as acceptance of living within this context.

In attentiveness meditation, one expands their conscious awareness. During meditation, you focus on what you experience, similar to the flow of your respiration. You can observe your own emotions and thoughts. However, allow them to pass without passing judgment.

Qi gong. Typically, this application incorporates meditation, relaxation, physical movement, and breathing exercises to restore and maintain equilibrium. vim gong (CHEE-gung) is an ingredient in traditional Chinese medicine.

Tai chi. This may be an application of light Chinese martial arts. In t'ai chi chuan (TIE-CHEE), you perform a self-paced series of postures or movements in a smooth, unhurried manner while engaging in deep breathing.

Transcendental meditation. Transcendental meditation could also be a straightforward and natural practice. During this type of meditation, you silently repeat an in-person assigned mantra, such as a word, sound, or phrase, in accordance with passing specific instructions. Without requiring concentration or effort, this type of meditation may enable your body to settle into a state of profound relaxation and your mind to realize a state of inner peace.

Yoga. You perform a series of postures and controlled breathing exercises in order to promote a flexible body and a calm mind. As you progress through poses that require balance and concentration, you are encouraged to focus more on the present and less on your hectic day.

Benefits Of Meditation

Meditation can give you a sense of calm, serenity, and equilibrium, which is beneficial to both your emotional and physical health. You can also use it to relieve tension and relax by refocusing your attention on something soothing. Meditation can teach you how to remain centered and maintain inner calm.

And these benefits continue even after your meditation session has concluded. Meditation can help you navigate your day with greater composure. And meditation may aid in the management of certain medical conditions' symptoms. Meditation is not a substitute for conventional medical care. However, it may complement your other treatment. Meditation and psychological and physical health

When you meditate, you may be able to eliminate the daily information overload that contributes to your tension.

Among the emotional and physical advantages of meditation are:

Obtaining a fresh viewpoint on stressful situations
Developing stress management abilities and increasing self-awareness
Present-mindedness Reduces negative emotions
Increasing inventiveness and originality
Increasing tolerance and forbearance
Reducing the heart rate at rest

Bringing down blood pressure at repose
Enhanced slumber quality
Mediation and disease

Meditation may also be beneficial if you suffer from a medical condition, particularly one that is exacerbated by tension.

While a growing body of scientific evidence supports the health benefits of meditation, some researchers believe it is not yet possible to draw definitive conclusions about the benefits of meditation.

In light of this, some research suggests that meditation may aid in the management of symptoms associated with conditions such as:

Anxiety
Asthma
Cancer
Chronic ache
Depression
cardiac disease
elevated blood pressure
Inflammatory bowel syndrome
Sleep concerns
Tension-related migraines

If you have any of the following conditions or other health issues, you should discuss the benefits and drawbacks of meditation with your doctor. In uncommon instances, meditation may exacerbate the symptoms of certain mental health conditions.

Having an Alpha Way of Life

After you have mastered the alpha male style and mentality, as well as the alpha male's healthy habits, you should implement the following daily adjustments to your lifestyle. These actions and behaviors will assist you in achieving long-term success and satisfaction in your personal and professional relationships. This is one of the few financial practices that Betas struggle to adopt.

Living a Life with Meaning

To qualify as an alpha male, one must be willing to undertake leadership responsibilities. His ability to achieve the ideal balance between politeness and assertiveness is the secret to his charismatic personality. This is a benefit in every situation. It may sound simple, but it is not always simple to implement.

Take one step at a time, and you will reach your destination. You can begin taking charge of your life in three easy actions.

Being an Effective Communicator – When a leader recognizes the positive qualities in others, those qualities are more likely to be utilized. This is essential to your professional and academic success. You will appear more approachable and likable if you never hurry to judgment. Over the next 30 days, make an effort to get to know your colleagues better by learning what makes them tick and encouraging them to play to their strengths.

Secondly, an alpha male is financially savvy. Another rule of dating etiquette is to always pay for the dinner of your companion. Consequently, you must ensure that you always have an emergency reserve set aside. For the next thirty days, save at least $10 per day by reducing expenses or acquiring additional income. When it comes to investments, it is also wise to invest in one's own education.

Despite the fact that domineering males are expected to intimidate both women and other men, they should always be humorous and gentlemanly. Being a gentleman can be demonstrated in every aspect of one's daily life. Only empathy and sincerity are necessary. There is nothing weak about offering an apology or acknowledging your errors. In reality, the opposite is true. Do something kind for someone every day for the next thirty days and observe their gratitude.

Consuming a Healthful Diet

You should know by now that alpha males maintain a healthy weight. Three meals per day are essential, but they are not the only factor. It is all about making food choices in accordance with your objectives. A caloric deficit is required for weight loss, which can be attained by consuming fewer calories than the body needs. When attempting to gain weight and being underweight, a caloric surplus is the opposite of a caloric deficit.

When dieting, how much you consume is more important than how frequently you eat. If you struggle to control your appetite, try consuming four to five small meals throughout the day. This will allow you to control your appetite throughout the day.

Defeating Your Doubts
Everyone on the planet experiences some form of anxiety or dread. When it comes to overcoming their anxieties, alphas are more intelligent than betas. Fears can be regarded either as a source of inadequacies or as a catalyst for development. In the next 30 days, do something you would normally be terrified of. It is essential that fears are not irrational, such as a dread of spiders, heights, or anything else that is counterproductive.
Never be afraid to attempt something new, whether it's starting a business, approaching a girl you like, or participating in a contest you've never entered before. As an alpha male, he

accepts these opportunities not only to increase his chances of victory, but also to enrich his existence.

The best method to boost your self-esteem and confidence is to believe you are an alpha male and to confront your fears head-on. As an illustration, if you have a fear of public speaking, set a goal to participate in speaking engagements and observe how comfortable you feel with your newly acquired self-confidence.

Encountering Your Greater Self

This is a guided meditation for meeting your higher self; you will learn how to communicate with your higher self, how to strengthen this connection, and how to receive invaluable advice. Your higher self is always with you; all you have to do is be still and tune in. With this connection, you will be guided to make the correct decisions in life and truly live for your highest good. So, to begin, focus on your breathing, inhaling deeply and slowly, allowing your stomach to expand as you inhale, and exhaling slowly as you feel your body relax. Once more, inhale and exhale slowly, allowing all tension to leave your body. Inhale and exhale, inhale and exhale, inhale and exhale, inhale and exhale.

Bring your focus to your feet; beginning with your toes, you can feel them becoming increasingly heavy as a wave of profound relaxation spreads throughout your entire body. This sensation travels from your feet, through your ankles, and into your lower legs like a magnificent light. Now, your feet, ankles, and lower legs feel extremely heavy and relaxed. As you unwind more and more, a feeling of absolute serenity spreads throughout your entire body. Feel this loving, warm sensation as it travels over your knees and into your thighs; you feel very calm, very relaxed, and very at ease; you can feel it as it slowly travels up your thighs, over your hips, and all the way up to your waist, and your body becomes progressively heavier. This sensation, this wavelike feeling, brings with it a sense of joy and profound tranquility as you become increasingly relaxed. You feel extremely heaviness, calmness, and relaxation.

This loving wave now travels up your chest, across your shoulders, and down your back; do you feel a profound sense of relaxation? The more this wave moves through you, the more profoundly relaxed you become as you float along to its beautiful dance of serenity throughout your entire body. This sensation is unlike anything you've ever experienced. Feel your body as it tingles and glows with the warmth of this loving sensation of peace and you feel so very heavy, so relaxed, so peaceful, but at the same time so light in your soul and mind, enjoy the experience, enjoy the amazing feeling of this peaceful calmness. This beautiful wave of love and peace now travels up your neck, over your head, and down your face, your eyes are relaxed, your nose, and your cheeks are so deeply relaxed and so very heavy that you cannot open your eyes even if you wanted to, they are so heavy, your mouth, tongue, and ears are so relaxed, so peaceful, so calm, and you can feel this wonderful sensation of deep peace as the wave continues to travel all over and throughout your body, you are so very calm now, so drows

This loving, calming, and gentle wave of energy continues to flow down your shoulders and arms to your elbows, assisting you to go deeper within yourself, to the most loving and peaceful place, your private place where no one can go but you, and reminding you that you are always safe, loved, and protected. Even your fingertips are relaxed as the wave of pure relaxation travels down through your wrists and into your hands. You are currently so relaxed that your entire body is at rest. Your entire body, mind, and spirit are very still, very heavy, and profoundly relaxed. Your body is so relaxed that even if you wanted to, you cannot move a single muscle, but that's okay because you don't want to. You feel as though you are one with nature, one with the world, and one with the cosmos; now, for a few moments, remain in this state of ecstasy, sustaining a sense of peace and harmony. Simply focus on your respiration and your heartbeat. Imagine that you are now surrounded by a magnificent white light, a genuinely brilliant light with numerous golden flecks shining throughout it. This is the light of protection, the light that keeps you safe on your journey to meet your highest self, can you see it? Now visualize roots growing out of the soles of your feet, see the roots going into the ground beneath you, see them as they push their way through the soil and you can hear the sound of thumping. This is the sound of your highest self calling to you. Now, firmly plant these roots deep within the earth itself; they are grounding you to Mother Nature herself.

Now you are on your own private island, walking along a well-trodden path; you see a fork in the path ahead and have the option of taking the left or right fork. The decision is yours to make. You proceed along your chosen path for a while, noticing the tall, elegant trees with their branches reaching up to the sky, and hearing the birds calling to one another as they fly high above you.

Can they be heard?

When you reach the conclusion of your chosen path, you see a large meadow filled with flowers of all types and hues. Notice how magnificent and detailed each flower is, notice the vibrant colors, you breathe in deeply and inhale all the different fragrances that surround you, breathe deeply as you walk slowly through your meadow filled with flowers, you notice the warmth of the sun on your face, it is comfortable and invigorating and you feel a gentle warm breeze as you walk along, as you are taking in the beauty of all your surroundings, you notice a few small insects flitting about. You are not afraid of them, nor are they afraid of you, and you sense that they accept your presence here. You see a massive ancient oak tree in front of you and you walk towards it. It's a very old tree, and you see a door within it with a large rust doorknob in the center. You see a room beyond and enter it; the room is large, uncomfortable, and decorated with numerous framed pictures. You observe them and realize that you recognize the person in them; it is you, from many different lifetimes and attired in many different fashions, but you still recognize yourself. Look at the images for a moment and really examine them.

You will walk to the opposite end of the room to a door, which you will open and enter to discover a beautiful, light, airy room with a table and two chairs. The room's design is up to you. Is it the twenty-first century, the eighteenth century, or the middle ages? Whatever feels appropriate to you, it's your room. You pull out your chair, take a seat, and wait. In your mind, ask your higher self to come to you, to come and be with you now. You feel the air around you begin to change; it almost becomes tangible; you could almost taste its density. Can you see the small, gorgeous, golden light hovering above the chair across from you as you sit?

This golden light grows larger and begins to take shape; you take a photograph, and as you watch while feeling very peaceful and calm, you observe that the form has evolved into the most magnificent creature you have ever seen. Its magnificence leaves you speechless; is this being male or female? what do they have on? What hue are their eyes? what hue is your hair? This beautiful being is your highest self, this beautiful being is who you truly are. You see a golden thread emanate from this being and grow towards you, and you watch without fear as it attaches to you. You are now fully connected to your higher self, and it feels as though this thread has always been there, because it has. You simply never noted it previously. Allow your mind to remain still and wait for any impressions, images, or words to enter. What message does your superior self wish to impart? You are welcome to pose a question. If you want an answer to something, you should pose the question. Your higher self communicates with you via words, images, or an instantaneous knowing. Therefore, sit for a while and get to know your highest self; ask any questions you desire; and take note of what you see and sense here. Be at harmony with yourself, communicate with yourself, and listen to find the answers you seek. It is now time to leave your higher self and return to the here unknown, so you stand up and thank your higher self for meeting with you, and you can feel the love coming from this amazing being of light, the love this being has for you is eternal, and the love that you have for yourself is eternal, and you feel so peaceful,so calm,so relaxed, and so very happy, and you turn and walk to the door and leave the room, and you walk back to the outer door. So, take a deep breath in and exhale slowly and gently, then take another deep breath in and exhale slowly and delicately again. When you are ready to bring your awareness back to your body, wiggle your fingers and toes.

Giving Up The Negatives

Negative thoughts and emotions can weigh heavily on the body and mind, causing unnecessary tension. It is essential to acknowledge these thoughts and emotions before releasing them.

Once the burden is lifted, you can replace the negative with the positive and rewrite your story to realize your full potential. You can access your inner peace, positive outlook, and capacity for self-healing by perusing this. I'm thrilled to offer you this hypnosis exercise to assist you in letting go of negativity and adopting a positive outlook in order to realize your maximum potential.

To begin, I invite you to make yourself comfortable, close your eyes if you wish, and settle progressively into relaxation. If it feels right, place your hands on your heart and verbalize the physical connection. Imagine breathing in light, love, and serenity into your heart as you inhale into your heart and its surrounding space. Visualize this light as you breathe it in; it is a vibrant, glowing light that, as you breathe it into your heart, fills your body with loving and grounding energy and warms it. As you continue to concentrate on your breath, inhale relaxation and exhale tension and constriction from the region surrounding your heart. Right now, choose to be fully present to this moment,to your experience as a whole, be present to your physical body, to the sounds around you and the surface below you, allow your arms to rest at your sides or in your lap if you prefer, as you continue to relax deeper and deeper, you can connect with yourself, if the idea resonates with you, choose to set the intention to open your heart today, open its flow of energy to welcome in love and light, to support you on your journey. With each inhalation, be receptive to the compassionate energy of the world around you, and with each exhalation, radiate that love. Allow this radiance of love to ground your energy and protect your energetic boundaries by visualizing and sensing this warm, glowing energy entering and filling your body before radiating out into the space around your body.

Allow your attention to linger on the energy emanating from your heart for a moment longer. Feel this energy as it expands and fills your entire body with love. Today, allow this state of comfort and relaxation to open your heart to the emotions and opportunities it will bring. You can experience tranquility when you let go of resistance and the tendency to force an outcome. Be willing to listen to your heart's messages without judgment or preconceived notions. Know that you are entirely supported and protected in this space today as you explore your heart's feelings. Take a moment to examine your entire body, beginning with your feet and moving very slowly up to your cranium. As each part of your body appears in your mind's eye. Scan for any areas where tension, tightness, or pain are common, or any areas where you sense the energy is stuck and not freely flowing. If there are areas of tension in your body, concentrate on that area for a moment and breathe the idea of a warm glowing light into it to soften it. This warm loving light will melt the tension away from your body, allowing you to relax completely. It will enable your entire body's energy to circulate freely. Feel yourself soften and let go as you continue scanning your body with a relaxed awareness. Feel this loving energy move throughout your entire body as it takes you deeper and deeper into a safe, supported state of relaxation. During the next moment of silence, continue scanning your body and bringing loving, relaxing energy to every part of your body.

And now that you are in a safe and comfortable state of relaxation, imagine that you are standing at the top of a beautiful white marble staircase, see the staircase in vivid detail, and rest your hand on the smooth, cool marble banister that runs along the side of the staircase. As you look down the staircase, you notice that there are 10 steps leading down; these are the steps that will lead you deeper into relaxation. You may now grasp the beautiful handrail and descend the stairs leisurely and safely as I count to three. You are so profoundly relaxed that you can feel the tension melting away, and you have completely let go of any responsibilities or tasks so that you can focus on yourself. (8) You enable your body and mind to become completely relaxed and tune out the outside world. This phase facilitates a deeper state of relaxation. You are dedicated to taking your life and aspirations to the next level. (5) As you descend, you experience the familiar sense of bodily liberation and mental clarity that accompany this state of relaxation. As you unwind more, you notice a light at the bottom of the stairs. (2) You continue deep into relaxation and (1) until you reach your deepest state of relaxation at the bottom of the staircase; at this point, you are entirely relaxed and at ease.

Take a moment to examine your environment in this dream; you can see more clearly now that the light is emanating from behind the door at the bottom of the staircase. This light is seeping out of the door's margins, expanding its illumination while being partially obstructed by the door. You have the impression that behind this door rests all of your capabilities and inner potential. This light is shining out only partially, allowing only a portion of your potential to be seen. The door is effectively blocking the light of your potential from being fully seen. You are aware that before this door can be fully opened, there are things you must let go of and obstacles you must remove. Recognizing that there are obstacles that must be released is the first step; take a moment and then release any negativity you may be holding onto; this negativity does not need to be named specifically; simply release it. Visualize the energy of negativity and the weight of limiting beliefs wafting away like a feather carried by the wind, only to be replaced by new positive beliefs. These limitations we impose on ourselves can prevent us from progressing toward our ideal existence and achieving contentment. Let it all go, let go of any expectations you have of yourself and any expectations you perceive others have of you, let go of the desire to please anyone other than yourself and the tendency to care what others think. Let go of attachments, let it all go, let go of competition with past versions of yourself and with others, let go of the idea of being perfect and the need to always be right, let go of the times when you find yourself thinking you should be saying or doing something in your life, let it all go, let go of excuses, let go of judgmental thoughts, let go of jealousy and thoughts of not being enough, let go of your insecurities, let it all go, let go of

Permit the past to be the past and not determine your future, and let go of anything else that is no longer serving you; be here now, be present, be mindful, be grateful, be joyful, and be love. Once all of these ideas, thoughts, and blocks have been released, begin to replace them with positive thoughts and energy. You can now replace these thoughts with the simple and powerful notion that you are enough. When you truly believe that you are enough, you will experience a profound sense of inner confidence and peace. Hear the words, sense them in your heart, and allow them to permeate your subconscious beliefs: you are sufficient.

Being enough means being comfortable with your body as it is today, being enough is being comfortable with what you have accomplished and what you have yet to accomplish, being enough means self-acceptance, and it is something we can all say to ourselves more often. Let this feeling of sufficiency settle into your belief system for a moment longer, let it sink into your body like muscle memory; what you put out into the world will return to you; put out positivity, send out love and light, radiate this positive energy outward to the world, and it will return to you. Now that you have let go of all the negativity and replaced it with positive love and light, you know it is time to open the door at the bottom of the staircase all the way, you know it is time to let the light, your light shine out all the way so you can live your fullest potential with a deep inner confidence and knowing that you are enough.

As you place your hand on the doorknob and pull, your inner strength, determination, and potential flow out, filling your mind and the space around you. Feel the strength and positivity flow out of your mind and into your entire body and heart. You have the space to fill up with your full potential, and you know that you are capable of achieving great things now that your inner strength and potential have been released from behind this door. As you step into this light, you can feel the energy and strength of your full potential surrounding you and filling you up; this energy increases your competence and motivation. You find a bench on the other side of the door where you can sit and contemplate your complete potential. With your newfound energy, confidence, and motivation, you allow your mind to wander and be creative. You allow yourself to be open to possibilities, you are open to change and the opportunities it brings, and you choose to soften into these possibilities with affection.

Although you have a strong sense of what you want and what is important to you, you are willing to give a little and be flexible. You understand that it takes time for changes to occur and take root. You are patient and grateful for where you are on this journey. You know you are exactly where you are supposed to be right now. While this isn't always simple, you are committed to doing what is in your best interest and in alignment with your values rather than what is simple. You also recognize that with change comes a variety of emotions, which you seek to feel, understand, and embrace without becoming attached to the outcomes. Repeat after me: I am open to change, I am deserving of affection and success, I am confident, and I work diligently toward achieving my goals. I believe in myself and my abilities, I am courageous and brave, I am authentically me, I am creating my own future, I follow my ambitions with passion and certainty, I let go of the past and concentrate on the present, I am sufficient, and I am thankful for today. You leave the bench, confident and at ease, and return through the doorway to the bottom of the stairs. As you stand at the bottom of the staircase, you are confident in your ability to accomplish anything you set your mind to. You recognize that you are capable of achieving your goals and have the potential to accomplish amazing things.

Everyday Meditation

Regularly incorporate meditation into your daily life. Meditation is not limited to a particular structure; it can be practiced at any time during daily life. No matter how long you endure, you will be a huge aid. Each day is an ideal opportunity for meditation because your mind is unaffected by the day's stress and anxiety. However, it is best not to begin meditation immediately after eating, as you may experience genuine discomfort, which will divert your attention.

Take a coach-led meditation course to enhance your skills. Consider enrolling in a meditation course taught by an experienced instructor if you feel you need additional guidance. You can search online for various meditation classes. Local fitness centers, resorts, schools, and concentrated meditation habitats offer classes in a variety of disciplines. You can also find numerous instructional videos about meditation on YouTube. For a more visceral experience, you can participate in an otherworldly retreat, during which you will devote days or even weeks to meditation.

You can also utilize various meditation applications to help you get things moving. The Knowledge Clock application provides free meditation guidance, allowing you to select the desired duration and level of guidance.

Read insightful books. Certain individuals believe that reading otherworldly books and rigorous sacred writings can help them delve deeper into meditation and acquire genuine tranquility and otherworldly consciousness. Books that are suitable for use as presentations include "Quintessence of Individual Reality" by Jane Roberts, "New Earth" by Eckhardt Toler, and "Brief Care" by Donald Altman. If you so desire, you can also extract some insightful proverbs or illustrative texts and review them the next time you meditate.

Utilize caution in day-to-day life. Meditation is not limited to your training sessions. You can also practice compassion in your everyday life. Simply concentrating on what is occurring in the inner and outer worlds at a particular time can have an effect. For instance, when you feel anxious, try to concentrate on your breath for a few moments to remove any negative thoughts or emotions from your perspective. You can practice mindfulness while dining by focusing on the food and all of your emotions. Attempt to be mindful of your body's changes and how you feel while performing any activity of daily life, whether sitting at a computer or sweeping the floor. This level of consideration and awareness is the pinnacle of life objectives.

Try practicing meditation in order to improve your ongoing mindfulness. Meditation is a technique that facilitates the practice of mindfulness in daily life. You should simply concentrate on particular elements of your environment or specific bodily sensations. For instance, you may concentrate on the blue pen or envelope on the table in front of you, or become more aware of your feet on the floor or your hand on the armrest of the chair. If you feel distracted, occupied, or under pressure, you may want to try this method. You can also endeavor to simultaneously focus on a variety of emotions. Focus on the key, the inclination of your hand, and, remarkably, the smell of metal when you receive the keychain.

Choose a sound lifestyle. Even though meditation can improve your overall health, it is more effective when combined with other healthy practices. Eat as healthily as possible, engage in more physical activity, and get sufficient rest. Prior to meditating, try to watch less television, don't smoke, and don't consume alcohol, as these behaviors impair the mind and are incompatible with clear cognition required for effective meditation.

You must recognize that meditation is a journey. Meditation is not a specific goal that can be accomplished, like advancement. It should be regarded as a tool to achieve your goals (regardless of whether your goal is "enlightenment"), similar to "going out" to realize "the world is so vast." You should concentrate on the interaction and experience of meditation, rather than bringing your day-to-day desires and relationships into your meditation practice. Beginning meditators should not focus excessively on the essence of meditation. It is considered a success if you feel more settled, happier, and tranquil after training for any length of time.

HINT

It is not difficult to ignore time during meditation, but doing so will only serve to distract you. Certain individuals believe that setting a warning can assist in resolving this issue, but be sure to select a warning with a softer ringtone. If the warning sound is excessively unexpected, you will be irritated by the possibility of constantly pondering when the alert sounds.

Focus on your emotions and thoughts on purpose when you are not contemplating. You will discover that on days when you are contemplating, you are more peaceful, joyous, and aware than on days when you are not. Try to prevent your internal voice from entering your psyche. You can fixate on these thoughts, but don't let them guide your actions.

If you want to meditate but feel exhausted, sore, exhausted, or otherwise unsuited to achieve a specific level of relaxation, then perform some relaxation exercises first. You can walk, run, take a shower, or do your chores first; these exercises can actually reduce stress. From that point forward, endeavor to recommence meditation.

Correct posture can create more space for the lungs and facilitate smoother respiration. In actuality, the overwhelming majority of the muscles from the hip to the neck are concentrated on the respiratory muscles of the stomach. You can sense that they are assisting the stomach relax, albeit only slightly. If you recognize this, your position is correct. The correct stance is simple to maintain and completely agreeable; you will feel as though you are floating on the water.

In perfect harmony, you can accomplish anything. Others merely enjoy the rare "rest" that meditation provides. Meditation is a means for individuals with strong religious convictions to communicate with their god(s) and attain enlightenment.

Meditation exerts its influence before the meditator learns how to fully concentrate or calm the mind. Meditation can be advantageous through simple practice. Select the strategy that best fits your needs. If the method that works for others does not work for you, do not give up without a fight. Keep in mind, decompress!

Haste is insufficient. Meditation does not produce an adept in Taoism overnight. Only pure meditation devoid of utilitarianism can produce the finest results.

Some of the advantages of inconspicuous meditation include the ability to fall asleep more easily, increased irritability, and changes in mindset (especially noticeable in Buddhists who meditate for over 1,000 hours). If you find it difficult to adhere to the meditation time you set, begin with a shorter meditation. Almost everyone can meditate for one to two minutes without becoming irritated by interruptions.

Then, after the waves subside, endeavor to extend the meditation period slightly until you can complete the entire process.

The benefits of long-term meditation are self-evident, and your perseverance is rewarded. These benefits include practicing awareness, reducing stress and negative emotions, enhancing memory and concentration, and increasing the amount of gray matter (synapses) in all parts of the mind.

The Musicians Of Bremen

A specific man had a jackass who had tirelessly transported maize sacks to the plant for the better part of a year; however, his loyalty was deteriorating and he was becoming increasingly unfit for work. Then his lord began to consider how he could best save his castle, but the jackass, observing that there was no reasonable wind, took off and set sail for Bremen. "There," he concluded, "I can unquestionably be a town performer." After a distance of walking, he discovered a dog lying in the open, wheezing as if he had run himself to exhaustion. "What are you heaving for, you massive individual?" questioned the cretin.

"Okay," the dog replied. "Since I'm old, growing weaker every day, and can no longer chase, my lord wanted to kill me, so I fled. However, how am I going to get food now?"

"I pause for a moment," said the cretin. "I'm going to Bremen and will be a town performer there; accompany me and establish yourself as an artist as well. You will play the kettledrum while I play the lute."

The dog agreed, and they continued on.

In a short time, they came upon a cat sitting on the road with a visage like three windy days! The imbecile inquired, "At this time, old shaver, what have you abandoned?"

"Who can be happy when his neck is in danger?" questioned the cat. "Since I'm currently declining, my teeth are worn down to stumps, and I prefer to stay by the fire and twist as opposed to chasing mice, my lover wanted to suffocate me, so I fled. In any event, sage advice is scarce at present. Where should I go?"

"Join us in Bremen. You understand nighttime music; you could be a city performer."

The cat appreciated it and followed them. Following this, the three outlaws arrived at a ranch yard where a chicken was seated at the entrance and crowing loudly. The stallion said, "Your crow is a complete one." "What is wrong?"

"I have been anticipating fine weather since it is the day Our Woman washes and dries the Christ-child's little shirts," said the chicken. "However, Sunday visitors are coming, so the housewife has no pity, and has informed the cook that she expects to eat me in the soup tomorrow, and tonight I'm to have my head cut off. Presently, I'm crowing as loudly as I can."

"Okay, but red-brush, you would be wise to leave us," said the jackass. You have a decent vocal, and if we make music together, it ought to be of high caliber!"

This arrangement was accepted by the poultry, and the four continued together. Nonetheless, they were unable to reach the city of Bremen in a single day, and they intended to spend the night in a nearby forest. The jackass and the dog laid down beneath a massive tree, while the cat and the chicken settled into the branches. However, the rooster flew directly to the summit, where he was generally safe. Before he fell asleep, he scanned the area from all four sides and believed he spotted a light, so he yelled to his companions that a home must be nearby because he saw the light. The jackass stated, "Assuming this is true, we'd be wise to move on, as the safe house here is terrible." The dog believed that a couple of bones with flesh on them would suffice.

They proceeded toward the source of the light and, as they approached, saw it grow brighter and larger until they reached a well-lit home for thieves. As the finest, the jackass went to the window and peered inside.

"What do you see, my dark pony?" the rooster questioned. The jackass was asked, "What do you see?" The jackass replied, "I see a table laden with food and drink, surrounded by looters having a good time." "That would be right up our alley," the poultry said. Indeed, certainly; oh, how I wish we were there!" remarked the idiot.

The animals then discussed how they could repel the intruders, and they eventually came up with an arrangement. The jackass was to place his front feet on the window sill, the dog was to jump on his back, the cat was to shift onto the canine, and finally the rooster was to fly up and roost on top of the cat.

At the point when this was completed, at a predetermined signal, they began to play their music together: the jackass whinnied, the dog barked, the cat meowed, and the rooster crowed; then they erupted through the window into the room, causing the glass to shake! At this dreadful commotion, the robbers leapt to their feet, convinced that a ghost had entered the building and fled in terror into the forest. The four friends sat down at the table, content with what was left, and consumed as if they were going to fast for a month.

When the four entertainers were finished, they turned off the lights and searched for a place to rest based on their individual preferences and needs. The jackass laid down on some straw in the yard, the dog behind the front door, the cat on the hearth close to the warm ashes, and the rooster roosted himself on a light emission rooftop; and, exhausted from their long trek, they soon fell asleep.

At the point when it was past 12 p.m., and the robbers saw from a distance that the light in their home had been extinguished, and everyone appeared calm, the captain said, "We ought not have allowed ourselves to be frightened out of our minds," and requested that one of them investigate the home.

The courier went into the kitchen to light a candle, mistaking the cat's flaming pupils for live coals and holding a lucifer match to them. However, the cat did not understand the jest and flew in front of him, spitting and scratching. As he ran across the yard to the bale of straw, the jackass kicked him in the rear with its hind foot. The rooster, agitated and energised by the pandemonium, yelled from the column, "Chicken a-doodle-doo!"

Then, the thief returned to his leader as quickly as he could and reported, "Ah, there is a terrible witch sitting in the house, who spat on me and scratched my face with her long paws; and by the entryway stands a man with a blade, who cut me in the leg; and in the yard lies a dark beast, who beat me with a wooden club; or more, on the rooftop, sits the appointed authority, who shouted, "

After this, the house no longer inspires confidence in the burglars; however, it fits the four Bremen performers so well that they do not wish to depart. In addition, the mouth of the last person to recount this story is still warm.

BENEFITS OF VIPASSANA

Know one's genuine personality

Self-liberation, a state of complete awareness and realization of one's true self, is the greatest advantage of Vipassana. According to Vipassana teachings, awareness of one's true nature arises when one stills the mind and transcends the ego's attachment to the physical world, including one's current identity and physical body. As you let go of these attachments, you gain the ability to recognize the truth of your being and essence, which is unconditional pleasure, bliss, love, and light.

The capacity to maintain composure
Vipassana teaches you to maintain equanimity regardless of your circumstances. Accepting all outcomes, positive or bad, with equanimity. Therefore, when you have a pleasant experience, you do not develop an attachment to it. Likewise, you do not avoid negative experiences when they occur. Being equanimous involves accepting all circumstances as they are. This practice promotes serenity and enables individuals to observe stressful situations without becoming emotionally involved.

Develop mental discipline and concentration
Vipassana encourages you to cultivate a sharp concentration on the tip of your nose and your breath. When your mind wanders, you return your attention to

your breathing. By consistently employing this method, you will develop mental strength and discipline. You will realize that we are rarely genuinely focused during the events of daily life. By focusing on this concentration, however, you improve your ability to think and see clearly.

Enhanced productivity over time

The enhanced self-awareness, discipline, and focus enable you to slow down and listen. The average human reportedly has 6,000 thoughts per day. But how much of that is mental white noise? Vipassana will enable you to concentrate on what is essential and disregard everything else. Being present and attentive enables greater concentration when performing duties. Which results in quicker and more efficient task completion.

Enhance physical well-being

When considering the health benefits of meditation, many people only consider the mental health benefits, ignoring the profound physical benefits meditation has on the body. Vipassana is particularly effective for this. When participating in a Vipassana course or retreat, practitioners are advised to adopt a plant-based diet and reduce their evening caloric intake.

New meditators are advised to snack lightly on fruit instead of consuming dinner, whereas experienced meditators are advised to eliminate all meals after noon.

Even at the earliest meals, a reduced diet is advised. All of this leads to improvements in physical health, including weight loss, the reduction of chronic disorders, and a decreased risk of cardiac disease.

In addition, Vipassana and the results of its practice have reduced detrimental cravings and addictions in a number of individuals, including but not limited to pornographic, alcohol, and smoking addictions.

Discover genuine, unconditional happiness

Alongside the sense of inner calm that Vipassana imparts is an undeniable sense of happiness or joy. This happiness is one of the primary objectives of Vipassana practice. Initially, achieving this state can take some time, but with practice, individuals can access their inner pleasure on command.

Basic Meditation Techniques

After preparing a silent, comfortable space and a comfortable seated position, you can begin to investigate various meditation techniques. You can attempt the following basic meditation techniques:

The respiration awareness technique The body scan technique The meditation of loving-kindness

The breathing awareness method
The breath awareness technique is a simple and accessible form of meditation that involves concentrating on the breath. It can help to calm the mind and promote relaxation, and is a useful starting point for people who are new to meditation. Here's how to practice respiratory awareness:

Finding a comfortable seated position is the initial phase of practicing the breath awareness technique. This may involve sitting on a cushion on the floor, sitting in a chair with your feet securely planted on the ground, or sitting with your legs crossed. Find a position that is comfortable, stable, and allows you to sit for extended periods of time without experiencing discomfort or pain.

➤ Concentrate on the breath: Once you are comfortably seated, direct your attention to the breath. Become aware of the sensation of the respiration as it enters and exits the body. Concentrate on the sensation of breath in the nostrils or the rising and falling of the thorax or abdomen.

➤ It is natural for the mind to wander during meditation, and this is perfectly acceptable. Whenever your mind wanders, simply return your focus to your inhalation. This can help to calm the psyche and promote clarity and concentration.

Continue for several minutes: The breath awareness technique can be practiced for as long as you like, but it's generally advised to begin with a few minutes and increase the duration of your practice gradually over time. You can use a timer to keep track of the practice's duration, or you can simply let it end spontaneously.

Overall, the breath awareness technique is a straightforward and efficient method to begin a meditation practice. By meditating on the breath, the mind can be calmed and relaxation achieved.

The body scan method
The body scan technique is a meditation technique that involves lying down and focusing on various areas of the body individually. This technique can aid in promoting relaxation and relieving muscular tension. Here's how to perform a body scan:

Lie on your back comfortably: The first stage in practicing the body scan technique is to lie on your back comfortably. This can be done on a yoga mat, a cot, or any other comfortable surface. Ensure that you are sufficiently toasty and won't be interrupted for the duration of your practice.

➢   After achieving a comfortable position while lying down, the next stage is to focus on your feet. As you focus on your feet, take a few long breaths and observe any sensations or emotions that arise. Do not attempt to alter anything; instead, observe and accept the status quo.

➢   After focusing for a few minutes on your feet, the next stage is to move your attention, one body part at a time, up the body. This may involve concentrating on your ankles, calves, thighs, etc., until you reach the top of your cranium. As you move your awareness through the body, take several deep breaths and become aware of any sensations or emotions that arise.

When you are ready to conclude your meditation session, take a few long breaths and open your eyes gradually. Observe any shifts in your mood or mental state and incorporate any insights or observations into your daily life.

The body scan technique is a basic and effective method for promoting health.

Compassionate meditation
The loving-kindness meditation is a technique for cultivating emotions of self- and other-compassion. This method can assist in fostering a sense of connection and compassion. Here is how to practice the meditation of loving-kindness:

The first step in practicing the loving-kindness meditation is to sit comfortably in a peaceful, comfortable environment. This can be done on a floor cushion, in a chair with your feet securely planted on the ground, or in any other comfortable seated position. Find a position that enables you to sit for extended periods of time without experiencing discomfort or pain.

➢ Bring a loved one to mind: Once you are seated comfortably, the next step is to recall a loved one. This could be a member of your family, a close friend, or anyone who fills you with feelings of affection and warmth. Repetition of loving-kindness phrases such as "may you be happy, may you be healthy, and may you be at peace" while thinking of this individual.

➢ After focusing on someone you adore, recall someone you are neutral toward. This could be a stranger, a casual acquaintance, or anyone who does not evoke strong sentiments of affection or aversion. Repeat the phrases of loving-kindness to this individual as you think of them.

➢ Finally, recall a person with whom you have conflict. This could be someone who has wronged you or someone with whom you have conflict. As you consider this person, repeat the loving-kindness phrases to them as well. This step's objective is not to attempt to alter your feelings toward this individual, but rather to foster a sense of compassion and understanding.

The loving-kindness meditation is a highly effective method for fostering a sense of connection and compassion. By routinely practicing this technique, you can cultivate a more accepting and loving attitude toward yourself and others.

There are numerous advantages to meditating, including:

Meditation has been shown to aid in the reduction of stress and anxiety by promoting relaxation and calming the psyche.

Meditation can enhance mood and overall sense of well-being by increasing the brain's production of feel-good chemicals.

Meditation helps improve focus and concentration by training the mind to remain in the present moment and resist distractions.

Research has demonstrated that meditation can help reduce blood pressure by relaxing the body and reducing tension.

Meditation can enhance the quality of sleep by calming the mind and promoting relaxation.

Several studies have demonstrated that meditation can strengthen the immune system by reducing stress and fostering relaxation.

Meditation has been demonstrated to improve cardiovascular health, including reducing the risk of heart disease.

Meditation can increase self-awareness by focusing one's attention on the present moment and cultivating clarity and comprehension.

instructions for Mindfulness meditation

Mindfulness meditation is a form of meditation that involves drawing one's awareness in a nonjudgmental manner to the present moment. It is a simple yet effective practice that can help reduce tension and enhance well-being overall.

Here is an overview of how to practice mindfulness meditation:

Find a peaceful, comfortable spot where you will not be disturbed where you can recline or lie down.

Close your eyes and take several deep breaths to calm your mind and body.

Focus your attention on the sensation of air entering and exiting your body as you breathe.

When your mind wanders, gradually return your focus to your breathing.

As you continue to concentrate on your breathing, observe your thoughts and emotions as they arise. Observe them without judgment and allow them to pass without becoming entangled in them.

If external stimuli distract you, simply acknowledge them and return your focus to your inhalation.

As long as you feel comfortable, continue to concentrate on your breath and the present moment, allowing your mind to become still and your awareness to expand.

It is essential to remember that mindfulness meditation is a practice that requires time and perseverance to develop. It is normal for the mind to wander, which is acceptable. The objective is not to eliminate all thoughts, but rather to become more aware of them and allow them to pass without becoming entangled in them. You will become more adept at returning your focus to the present moment and experiencing a sense of inner calm and clarity with practice.

What does the practice of meditation entail?
If tension causes you to feel tense, restless, and uncomfortable, try meditating. You can regain your equanimity and tranquility with only a few daily meditation sessions. Meditation is a practice that can be performed by anyone. It is simple and inexpensive. And standard instruments are adequate for the job.

The history of meditation is extensive. The original purpose of meditation was to gain mental insight. To become acquainted with it. As a means of relaxing and de-stressing, a growing number of people turn to meditation today.

Meditation, considered an alternative remedy for the mind and body, is gaining popularity. Meditation is capable of inducing a profound sense of peace and tranquility. The purpose of meditation is to train the mind to be more attuned to the experience of the present moment and to free it from the racing, chaotic thoughts that can be a source of tension. The technique may enhance an individual's mental and physical health.

As a form of stress relief, meditation can assist you in processing the immense amounts of information that accumulate daily in your brain.

Why teach infants mindfulness?
Finding methods to help children and their families relax their bodies and minds is crucial in today's hectic world. But tranquility alone is insufficient; awareness is also necessary.

Meditation is an excellent method to relax the entire body. This has consequently beneficial effects on the mind, body, and spirit. In particular, mindfulness meditation is acquiring popularity as a method of disease prevention and treatment.

Several studies conducted in educational settings have also demonstrated improved concentration and behavior. In studies involving individuals with ADD/ADHD, stress, anxiety, poor academic performance, insomnia, disruptive conduct, and eating disorders, benefits were reported. In a study involving 300 modern, low-income, minority middle-schoolers, school-based mindfulness education improved mental health and decreased post-traumatic stress disorder (PTSD) symptoms.

A reduction in stress hormones and a tranquil effect on the nervous system are physiological benefits. Scientific studies have demonstrated benefits for digestive issues, obesity, migraines, hypertension, pain perception, and immune function. As an illustration, a study of 166 high-risk adolescents revealed that they were able to reduce their blood pressure and pulse rate during meditation by simply becoming more aware of their respiration.

Curiosity and inquisitiveness come naturally to infants. They have a desire for knowledge, a fascination with the present, and the ability to pay careful attention. Similar to adults, children are frequently preoccupied. They are exhausted, readily influenced, and agitated. Too many children today lack sufficient leisure to "be" or do nothing. They develop quickly. Young people are frequently required to juggle multiple roles outside of the classroom. With everything else that students must study and memorize, this rapidly becomes overwhelming. The query is why they appear to be perpetually active with no option to pause them.

When children engage in mindfulness practices, they are taught to take a deep breath, center themselves, and identify their immediate requirements. They are able to cease acting on autopilot, recognize their impulses, and accept that not everything is perfect.

They have learned to create a nice scene wherever they go. They develop the ability to be internally and externally frank and transparent about their lives. Your children will flourish in an environment that provides them with the care, tolerance, confidence, and understanding they require to develop their individual personalities.

At what age do infants begin to benefit from mindfulness practices?
Mindfulness practice can help children as young as seven to calm their racing thoughts, gain insight into their emotions, and enhance their concentration. In addition, they are suitable for children with low self-esteem who need reassurance that it's okay to be themselves.

Numerous adolescents have low self-esteem and are concerned that they do not measure up. They worry, then react with their distorted sense of self by isolating themselves or desiring attention, by attempting to please others or placing themselves first, by being aggressive or tough. They are unable to break out of unproductive for their development regimens.

Nevertheless, the overwhelming majority of young people enjoy and benefit from physical activities. Even though meditation is not therapy in the traditional sense, it can be quite useful in helping children cope with difficult emotions and impulses that they might otherwise act on without pausing to consider the consequences.

Third Chapter: Practical Energy Work

How to Detect Energies

Sensing energy is a skill that requires practice to master. Although you can see and hear with your eyes and hearing, respectively, there is no specialized organ for sensing energy. How specifically do you make it function? You must maintain an open and focused mind in order to detect energy.

All things are energy. You have both external and internal energy. The difficulty is that it is much simpler for you to perceive the energy within your own body, given that it is your own body, but with practice you can expand your perceptive abilities to encompass other entities.

Therefore, it is better to start with you. In addition to using your hands to sense yourself, you can also use your inner awareness to perceive what is occurring within you. Simply direct your attention to whichever region of your body you wish to focus on. You should begin with your hands because they are the most sensitive to energy.

Stand or sit as comfortably as possible while maintaining a straight spine.

Maintain your palms at chest level, two inches apart, and at chest level. You should have your palms facing each other.

Consider your hands, direct your awareness or focus to your palms, and observe the distance between them.

As you inhale, gently draw your palms apart from one another.

Exhale as you bring your hands back together.

Maintain your respiration and hand movements while focusing gently on your palms and the space between them as it changes. You may experience cold, heat, pressure, electricity, tingling, or lightness, as well as a magnetic push and draw. These sensations represent your expanding consciousness of energy.

When minutes have passed, release your hands and take three deep breaths in and out.

The Way to Make an Energy Ball

If you have ever needed an energy boost without the jitters caused by your favored coffee, you should learn how to make energy balls. It is even greater than energy because you can use it to improve your manifesto. A orb of energy is composed of energy, also known as prana or chi if you prefer.

You can use an energy ball to restore your vitality when you feel exhausted. If you're feeling a little under the weather, you can use an energy orb to feel better. Using the energy orb, you can heal your pet if they are unwell. Want security? Create an orb of energy and envelop yourself in it. Additionally, energy spheres can draw you closer to divine beings. Best of all, they are fantastic for accelerating manifestations.

Energy balls are literal spheres of energy that are formed by the hands. You have already gained expertise with this through a previous exercise. There are chakras on each forearm, allowing you to generate this energy. When your palm chakras are balanced and open, you are comfortable receiving compliments because you have a strong sense of self-worth. You laud yourself for your extraordinary skills and abilities and do not criticize yourself. If you are a writer, the words come easily. You have no problem listening to others, even if they have a different opinion than you. When you enter a room, you immediately know whether you should be there or not. You have an intuitive notion of whether something is good or not.

How to construct an energy ball:

Find a place where you will not be interrupted and eliminate all distractions. Request to not be interrupted.

Focus on your respiration for a few minutes, or until you feel at ease, while seated in a comfortable position.

Imagine the energy as a beam of light emanating from the top of your cranium and penetrating the earth like tree roots. Imagine the earth's energy flowing through you.

Place your palms at chest level, with your palms facing each other and a few inches apart. If you prefer, you can also place one palm over the other while maintaining the distance between them.

Deeply inhale and exhale as you move your palms in a circular motion.

Visualize a white light orb forming in the center of your palms in your mind's eye. Feel its vitality and attractiveness.

As you move your palms, you will observe that they begin to move farther apart. This occurs because the spheroid is growing in size.

You can now program your intentions into the ball. Imagine it connecting with your solar plexus chakra and feel the energy flowing back and forth between the orb and this chakra in order to heal yourself.

If there is a painful area on your body, transfer the ball there with the intention of healing it.

Move the ball around your companion if they require healing or need to be calmed.

You can also visualize what you want to occur and then send the orb out into the world to do your bidding.

How to Detect the Chakras

Before you commence, be sure to consult the section on chakras to determine their proper placement.

Now, a companion is required for this. Allow them to recline down on a bed or massage table if you have one.

Keep your palms a few inches apart above their body.

Beginning just below the groin, slowly move your hands along the middle of their body, working your way up to their cranium. Check to see if, as you move your palms, you can detect a difference in energy where the chakras should be.

It is possible to see colors or images associated with the chakra, but it is more likely that you will simply sense the energy with your hands.

The capacity to perceive chakras varies from person to person. Some people sense heat, while others feel cold. Certain individuals feel a buzz in their palms. In any case, the greater your practice, the more adept you will become at sensing the chakras. It is acceptable if you cannot find the words to convey your emotions. At each chakra, one can perceive or experience something.

Certain chakras will provide you with more information than others, and you may sense an imbalance or a release. It depends on who you are dealing with and the circumstances of their existence. Do not allow yourself to become disheartened if you do not perceive anything. It is acceptable to envision sensing the chakras. Imagination will enable you to access your psychic powers. Lastly, do not permit yourself to be uncertain. As a general rule, if you believe you have detected something while practicing, you have. The greater your confidence in your abilities, the greater your progress.

Sensing Chakras Using a Pendulum

A pendulum is a small, heavy object suspended by a short chain or cord. It should ideally be something meaningful to you that you can appreciate visually, such as a crystal, stylized key, stone, or whatever else is significant. How to utilize it to perceive chakras:

Maintain the pendulum over your chakra. Ensure it drapes a few inches above this chakra. Wait until there is complete silence.

Following a brief delay, your pendulum will commence to swing.

When it moves clockwise, the chakra is functioning normally.

When it moves in a counterclockwise direction, the chakra spins in the opposite direction.

When the pendulum is completely still or only moves in small circles, this chakra's activity is minimal.

When the chakra moves in vast circles, its activity is excessively high.

The chakra is healthy when it moves in a moderate circle and in a clockwise direction.

Meditation for various purposes:

How to tailor your meditation practice to achieve specific objectives, such as reducing stress and anxiety, enhancing concentration and focus, and nurturing a sense of inner serenity and happiness.

Meditation is a flexible practice that can be adapted to accomplish a variety of specific objectives. Here are a few ways to customize your meditation practice to accomplish various objectives:

Try incorporating mindfulness meditation into your practice in order to reduce tension and anxiety. This involves focusing on the present moment and being objectively aware of one's thoughts and emotions. Other forms of meditation that may be beneficial for reducing stress and anxiety include loving-kindness meditation, which involves focusing on feelings of love and compassion, and transcendental meditation, which uses a mantra to relax the mind.

If you would like to improve your focus and concentration, consider incorporating focused attention meditation into your daily routine. This involves concentrating on a single object, such as the respiration, to prevent the mind from wandering. Mantra meditation and chakra meditation are additional forms of meditation that may be useful for enhancing concentration and focus.

Try incorporating loving-kindness meditation into your practice in order to cultivate a sense of inner peace and happiness. This involves cultivating sentiments of self-love and compassion for others. Mindfulness meditation and visualization meditation are additional forms of meditation that may be useful for cultivating inner calm and happiness.

You can tailor your meditation to accomplish specific goals and improve your overall well-being by incorporating various types of meditation into your practice and maintaining a consistent meditation routine. As you learn and develop, remember to be patient and kind to yourself, and to approach meditation with an open and inquisitive mind.

Meditation Is Natural To You

What do you mean by "meditating?" Is there a way to utilize this technique? Exists any form of labor involved? Would you describe it as a mental difficulty or an impossibility? Certainly not.

If thought is the only thing occurring, then whatever helps individuals meditate must be external to the mind, since thought cannot alter the external world. The mind cannot penetrate the stage of awareness that marks the beginning of meditation. Keeping this in mind is essential, as it is the source of all our actions. As soon as we turn our attention inward, however, we revert to a state of mind that is focused on actions and processes, having learned through experience that anything is possible with sufficient will and faith. Yes. The mind is capable of everything except meditation, and the mind can accomplish anything besides meditation. You do not need to "get" meditation because you already possess it. Knowing that someone is considering and remembering you is sufficient. If you follow the arrow, it will become accessible to you. You seem to carry it with you at all times.

Being a meditator is not an action; it is a state of being. Since there is no such thing as not having it, it is impossible to obtain. Simply put, such an entity does not exist. Indeed, it's you. It represents the core of your being.

Once meditation is understood, everything becomes obvious. You are not required to emerge from the shadows if you choose not to.

Meditation is not a disorder, but rather a state of tranquil concentration. Human cognitive processes are disorganized and jumbled. Never does a moment of lucidity occur. It simply lacks logic. You are surrounded by invisible clouds of mental activity when you are deeply contemplating. The cloud they generate impairs visibility. Clarity is achieved when you are not distracted by your own thoughts and can concentrate solely on the task at hand. Your vision becomes not only expansive but also penetrating, reaching deep into the center of your being.

Meditation is essential for clear vision. You would never consider the possibility. You lack the ability to speak. Just because I say "Stop thinking" does not imply that you should promptly draw conclusions. Unfortunately, I must use words to convey my meaning, so I implore you to "drop thinking," but if you do, you will fail because you will once again reduce it to an action.

Sit. The act of doing nothing is abbreviated as "drop thinking." Stop forcing yourself to relax your consciousness. Try not to force your thoughts out of your mind. You withdraw to the room's perimeter and remain there, staring at the wall. in a casual, natural manner. I am not in a rush to leave at the moment. It is as if your mind and spirit are peaceful and alert while your body falls into a deep slumber. While your intellect remains active, your body is resting.

If you do not attempt to organize your thoughts, they will find serenity on their own. What do you do with your time? similar to the silt that would clog a stream if it abruptly resumed flowing freely. You decide to venture into the water and begin the process of draining it. If you make matters worse by adding to the muck, it will be nearly impossible to move around. Relax and enjoy the ride. Okay, let's give it some additional time. There is no possibility of improvement. No matter what you do, the watercourse water will become more polluted. If you wait for the stream to recede before crossing it, you will avoid sinking into the muck and decaying leaves on the other side. Relaxing on the bank will help you forget about your concerns. Observe indifferently. As the stream continues to meander through the region, it will eventually settle to the ground, carrying the mud and dead leaves with it. After some time, the stream's water is as transparent as before.

Each time a new desire enters your consciousness, the water becomes increasingly murky. Please relax and take a seat. It is not worth endeavoring to repair. The Japanese practice of doing nothing but remaining still is known as zazen. Eventually, individuals begin meditating. It is not something you must actively pursue; it discovers you. You'll recognize it when it arrives; it's always been there; you just weren't searching in the right place. The money was always available, but you were preoccupied with a million other things: your ideas, your aspirations, etc. You were not considering the only thing that matters: yourself.

Buddha refers to this process of redirecting one's energy as parabvrutti, or returning one's vitality to its source; at this point, one experiences a sudden and poignant clarity. Then you might hear ancient music in the pines and see clouds from a thousand miles distant. You will then have access to everything.

There are mental fundamentals that must be mastered. Knowing how the mind operates increases the probability that you will leave it alone. To be able to sit in zazen, to simply sit, sit, and do nothing, to let meditation occur, you must have a solid understanding of how the mind functions. Additionally, something is occurring.

But it helps to know about the mind, because if you don't, you may continue to do things that keep the mind functioning, thereby giving it your assistance.

The mind is initially in a constant state of commotion. Whether you are conscious or asleep, there is always a quiet conversation occurring in your head. You could be driving or digging a trench in your garden while conversing with yourself. The intellect is perpetually in conversation.

If you can temporarily suppress your thoughts, you will experience no-mind. This is the substance of meditation. The optimal state is one of mindlessness. This is your nation. But how does one attain a state of mental silence? You will fail again if you attempt. Certainly, no effort is required. Actually, the pause occurs frequently; one must simply be attentive to observe it. In the same way that there is a delay between each mental process, there is also a pause between each utterance. If we do not keep our thoughts separate, our words will collide. Their territories differ from one another.

What you say is true: a rose is a rose is a rose.

You emphasize the letters "a" and "rose," but pay little attention to the comma that separates them. Take a different approach.

When the younger one is on display, the older one, which is always there but cannot be seen, is hidden.

The mind can only process one idea at a time, so dualistic thought is impossible.

Its poor reputation prevents tens of millions of people from enjoying its benefits. It appears to be a place where only the terminally ill, the always-sad, and those who have lost all sense of humor would feel at ease.

Focus on the gaps in conversation rather than the filler words.

The space between spoken words is the artist's canvas. Words come and go, but silence endures. When you first appeared on Earth, you were a blank slate, a chasm. You came with nothing, an infinite nothing, and then you began to collect words.

Because of this, it will be difficult for you to remember your past beyond the age of four.

You are nothing more than a lifeless shell.

I was told that Shankara used to tell a story about a student who asked his teacher repeatedly about the nature of the ultimate self, but the teacher ignored him until one day, when he turned to the student and said, "I am trying to instruct you, but you are not listening. Individuality is internal tranquility. "

The mind is where words are formed, but I am the silence itself. So, "self" may be understood in this context. You were born with it; it has never been absent.

Mantras are used to silence individuals one by one until they are unable to speak.

After the next turn, you'll reach a place of relative calm.

If language changes throughout time, as it always does, then learning a new language will never become old. Whether it's a new word, concept, idea, or even just a wish, novelty is always attractive. But if you discover that all you're doing is thinking over and over the same thing, you could just stop thinking altogether. The great majority of devotees who recite mantras often report feeling sleepy, which is something I am well aware of. For many centuries, it was also a distinct possibility. As any mother can tell you, this is common knowledge. The purpose of a lullaby is to help a child unwind and drift off to sleep with the soothing sound of music or a repetitive chant. Hearing the same two or three lines repeated over and over in monotone can make a child tired. There's nowhere for the kid to go, so if you keep repeating the same thing over and over again, he'll become bored and fall asleep. He instructs you to keep repeating, so do it. I think it's time for bed. Soon enough, he begins to drift off.

Because TM's mantra chanting is known to put its practitioners to sleep, it is often recommended for those with insomnia.

Keep in mind that you want boredom, not sleep, when adopting a mantra for this purpose. If it doesn't work, you're out of luck. It is imperative to avoid falling asleep. Repeat the phrase in your head and resist the urge to fall asleep.

P. D. Ouspensky, a well-known devotee of Gurdjieff, was dying. The doctors advised him to rest, but he disregarded their advice and instead walked all the way across the city until dawn. It was widely believed that he had gone insane. His strength was waning, and he felt helpless. He needed to stop walking immediately or hasten his own demise. However, he continued to walk.

What are you doing? asked someone.

He desired to die with his eyes open. If I die in my sleep, I won't be able to experience the beauty of passing away. He was walking peacefully to his grave when he abruptly passed away.

In Bodhgaya, the location where Gautama Buddha attained enlightenment, there is a small path leading to the vicinity of the bodhi tree. Buddha walked continuously along this street after meditating for an hour beneath the tree.

They would inquire as to why, and he would respond, "Because if I sit under the tree for too long, fatigue sets in."

If you begin to feel tired, get up and go for a walk; otherwise, you may fall asleep and nullify the effects of your chant. The goal is to bore yourself to the point of insanity so that you will leap over a precipice.

All Zen rites and rituals are repeated indefinitely. You may perform them while seated, but you should get up and move around if you feel sleepy. As soon as you realize you are no longer asleep, resume your meditation position.

Remember that your mind is always active and dependent on its constant discourse for survival; therefore, escape the confines of your own thoughts.

This could be accomplished by exerting more effort, but doing so would significantly reduce your chances of success.

If the current practice of keeping children in school for five or six hours per day is any indication, they will soon develop atrophied brains and lose interest in learning. Almost all of us will die without ever having tapped into our latent intelligence.

You think religious people are completely stupid, but your biases are preventing you from realizing this. However, if you take a good, hard look at your sannyasins, you will discover that they are completely devoid of any sign of intelligence or originality. Their actions have had severe consequences for India.

At one point, a concerned spouse revivalist cried, "Stand up, all you spouses!""

In the chapel, only one man was seated while the rest of the men stood.

Pastor exclaimed, "Ah!You are one-of-a-kind.

Despite his protests, the man was unable to rise to his feet. I can't think of a better way to communicate "I am paralyzed."

Lack of sleep is not a meditative state and has no positive effects on health.

Suggestions for maintaining your objectives

Once you've set your goals, it's important to remain on track and make progress toward achieving them. Here are some tips for staying motivated and focused:

Create a plan. Break down your goals into smaller, actionable stages and create a plan for achieving them. This will make your goals more manageable and provide you with a road map to follow.

Track your progress By regularly reviewing your goals and measuring your progress, you can remain motivated and see how far you've come.

Share your goals with a friend, family member, or accountability partner, and ask them to routinely check in with you on your progress. This will help to keep you accountable and motivated.

Celebrate your accomplishments. When you achieve a goal or make progress toward one, take a moment to celebrate and recognize your success. This will help you remain motivated and focused on your next objective.

Life is unpredictable, and sometimes things don't go as intended. Instead of becoming disheartened if you encounter setbacks or obstacles, be adaptable and modify your plan accordingly.

By adhering to these guidelines, you can remain focused and motivated while working towards your objectives.

The Benefits Of A Fresh Start

Beginning the new year with a clean slate can be an effective way to set new objectives, make positive changes, and improve your overall health. Among the advantages of a new beginning are: The opportunity to recalibrate and refocus. You have the opportunity to let go of the past when you start over. This can be an effective method for resetting and refocusing on what's crucial.

Enhancement of well-being. The ripple effect of making positive life changes can result in enhanced physical and mental health. By beginning anew, you can create new habits and routines that are more in line with your values and objectives, which can contribute to greater well-being overall.

Enhanced motivation and vitality. You can experience a renewed sense of purpose and motivation when you begin again. This can increase your energy levels and inspire you to make positive changes in your life.

Improved interpersonal relationships. Restarting can also be a great method to improve interpersonal relationships. By establishing new boundaries, acquiring new communication skills, or simply being more present and mindful, you can enhance your relationships with others and forge deeper bonds.

The opportunity to recalibrate and refocus, improved well-being, increased motivation and energy, and improved relationships are just a few of the advantages that can result from a fresh start in the new year.

The first of the seven major chakras is the root chakra. When you cleanse and heal your root chakra, you create a solid foundation for the higher chakras. Without a solid foundation, you cannot expect anything you build to be sustainable. Having a roof over your head and enough money to cover your basic requirements are associated with your root chakra, but the root's power extends far beyond that. It is equally important to meet your basic emotional requirements as it is to meet your survival needs.

It is possible to have a secure employment and still feel insecure. You can have a robust bank balance and still be financially concerned.

How secure you feel on a daily basis has little to do with your financial situation and more to do with how secure you felt as a child. The Jesuits claim that if you give them a child until he or she is seven years old, they will reveal the man. The first seven years of your existence are crucial and will have a lasting impact on you. In fact, many of us spend the ensuing years recovering from the experiences of our formative years. During these years, your root chakra is highly active, preparing you for the remainder of your life. If you were completely supported to feel safe and secure as a child and were able to trust your caregivers, you will carry this same sense of trust and security into adulthood. You will believe that the world will provide for your basic requirements and then some - and it does.

But if you were neglected, felt unloved, were surrounded by hostility and violence, or had caregivers who sometimes met your needs and sometimes ignored you, it may be difficult for you to feel secure as an adult, even if you have everything you need.

Symptoms of root chakra disharmony

Problems with the root chakra may manifest in numerous forms. You are unlikely to encounter all of these symptoms, but if you recognize some of them in yourself, you should consider working on your root chakra. An unbalanced root chakra could result in:

Issues with your digestive system, specifically your colon
Problems with your bladder or intestines
Lower back, limb, or foot pain or difficulties
Prostate problems if you're male
Eating disorders
Weight gain or metabolic issues may indicate a problem.
Money issues, such as debt and compulsive spending
Struggling to find or hold down a job
Difficulty in finding the right career
Aggression
Egotism
Lack of self-assurance
or lack of resolve
Depression
Feeling ungrounded
Compulsive or uncontrollable behavior
Greed

Trust issues

Obsession with material possessions at the expense of other aspects of one's existence.

Harmonizing the base chakra

Even if you don't perceive any issues with your root chakra, you should always begin your chakra exercises by concentrating on it. As previously discussed, the root is the basis for everything that follows. Ensuring that your foundations are solid will facilitate the free passage of energy through the other chakras.

Meditation is one of the most effective methods to release energy. This can be a spiritual practice, but it can also be extremely grounding for the root chakra. If you have trouble trusting that the universe will provide you with what you need, connecting to whatever higher power you believe in, be it God, Spirit, the Universe, Nature, or simply your Higher Self, and developing a loving, trusting relationship with that higher power will help you feel safe even when you're at a low point.

Usually, it is preferable to meditate while sitting upright. During meditation, our minds enter the slower, deeper brainwaves associated with sleep, and if we are too relaxed, we may find ourselves dozing off. Perhaps this is what our systems require! There is no judgment if you fall unconscious while meditating, but it is not meditation.

If you find yourself falling unconscious frequently during meditation, sit up. Sometimes a change in posture is sufficient to break the connection between slowing down and falling asleep. Try holding a pebble in your hand during meditation if that is not enough. If you begin to nod off, your hand will relax, allowing the pebble to fall to the ground, where it will create a noise and wake you up. Over time, you will learn to recognize the signs of approaching slumber and to rouse yourself from the verge of sleepiness.

My book, Peace From Within, is replete with advice and techniques to help you establish a meditation practice.

Before we begin the first meditation, I would like to say that not all meditations are suitable for everyone. Some meditation techniques will be effective for you, while others will not. Some will be simple, while others will be difficult. Some will be enjoyable one day and tedious the next. Therefore, I will provide you with multiple meditation techniques for each chakra, so you can determine which is best for you.

Although this is a form of meditation, meditation is not about eradicating all thought. When people tell me they can't meditate, I assume one of two things: either they don't comprehend what meditation is or they haven't found the right method.

Therefore, approach these meditations with an open mind and observe the results. If you're one of the roughly 10% of people who can't visualize, there's nothing wrong with you if you can't 'see' objects in your mind. It is simply the way your intellect is wired. Try another technique, such as meditative movement.

Let your experience be your experience. It's all a part of this journey we call existence.

You may find it useful to record yourself reading the scripts so that you can unwind and maintain your concentration in the moment. You can also access recordings of the meditations on my YouTube channel, Chakra Movement.

Meditation script – Embracing Trust

Go somewhere where you will not be interrupted and get comfortable. Maintain a supported back position throughout the duration of the meditation.

Close your eyes and concentrate on your breathing. Observe how it flows in and out naturally, without you having to exert any effort.

Your respiration is always present, sustaining and nourishing you.

Spend a minute or two connecting with the present moment by merely sitting with your breath.

Now, take a deep breath in and direct it to your feet. Release any tension you may be harboring in your body.

Repeatedly inhale profoundly, sending the healing breath to your feet. Release any tension that may be present.

Once more, inhale profoundly and allow your breath to flow down to your feet. Exhale any residual stress or tension.

Now, take a deep breath in and direct it to your legs. Release any tension you may be harboring in your body.

Repeatedly inhale deeply, sending healing breath down your thighs. Release any tension that may be present. Once more, inhale deeply and allow your breath to travel down your legs. Exhale any residual stress or tension.

Now, take a deep breath in and direct it to your pelvis and groin. Release any tension you may be harboring in your body.

Once more, inhale deeply and direct the healing breath to your pelvis and groin. Release any tension that may be present. Once more, inhale thoroughly, sending this breath down to your hips and groin. Exhale any residual stress or tension.

Now, take a long breath in and direct it to your abdomen. Release any tension you may be harboring in your body.

Repeatedly inhale deeply, sending the restorative breath to your abdomen. Release any tension that may be present. Once more, inhale profoundly and allow your breath to flow down to your abdomen. Exhale any residual stress or tension.

Now, take a deep breath and send it to your heart to fill it with affection. Send out love to the universe as you exhale.

Inhale deeply once more, sending the healing breath to your heart in order to fill it with even more affection. As you exhale, release your love into the universe.

Once more, inhale profoundly, filling your heart with so much love that it overflows. As you exhale, send this love throughout the world and into the cosmos.

Now, take a deep breath and direct it to your larynx. Release any tension you may be harboring in your body.

Repeatedly inhale thoroughly, sending the healing breath to your throat. Release any tension that may be present.

Repeatedly inhale profoundly, sending this breath down to your throat. Exhale any residual stress or tension.

Now, inhale thoroughly and fill your head with this breath. Release any anxiety or tension you may be holding in.

Inhale deeply once more and distribute the healing breath throughout your cranium. Exhale any anxiety or tension that may be present.

Inhale profoundly once more, sending this breath throughout your entire head. Exhale any remaining anxiety or tension. Now, allow your breath to return to its normal, natural course. Observe how much easier, more relaxed, and full of comfort it now feels.

Currently, everything is wonderful. Each moment is flawless. You can have faith that every moment serves your highest good. Always, you will be held by your oxygen. The universe will always hold you in its embrace.

To assist you remember this, we will repeat a mantra in silence. And this mantra is I have faith.

I have faith in the universe.

I believe in myself.

I have faith that everything works out for the best.

I have faith in this instant.

I believe.

I believe.

I believe.

Spend a few minutes repeating I trust to yourself in silence. I believe. I believe.

Let go of the mantra and dwell with yourself in the present moment. Observe how relaxed, tranquil, and supported you feel.

And if you ever experience feelings of uncertainty or doubt, you can return to this mantra and recite it to yourself. Recognize that everything will always turn out well in the end.

When prepared, you may open your eyes.

PART II: IMPROVING YOUR BODY
To be at your best, you must also take care of your body and be operating on all cylinders! Here are a few daily additions you can make to achieve this...

Deep respiration: Practice breathing deeply
Of course, if you cease breathing you die...I'm referring to deep respiration. 70% of your body's toxins are expelled via your lungs and exhalation, making "full breathing" a potent and natural detoxifier.

In his Ten-Day Challenge, peak-performance expert Tony Robbins recommends deep breathing. Three times per day, 10 "power breaths" are taken with a ratio of 1-4-2. If you inhale for six seconds, you will hold your breath for twenty-four seconds and exhale for twelve seconds.

This form of breathing energizes the body, thereby making it healthier and less stressed. You'll begin to feel better almost immediately...Try it out now. I'll wait.

Consume "productive" dishes
We've discussed a number of things you can do to increase your productivity, but did you know that the foods you consume can also help? That is correct. The foods you consume on a daily basis can affect how well your brain functions, making it simpler (or more difficult) to achieve your objectives.

According to research, your brain functions optimally when you consume a specific quantity of glucose (exactly 25 grams) that is released slowly over time. This category includes foods that have positive effects on the body and psyche, such as:

Fish Nuts Seeds
Avocado Blueberries
Raw carrots and...an almost universal favorite:
The darkest chocolate

Consume these nutrients, and your body and mind will thank you.

Drink more water: 9-13 glasses a day
Nearly 75 percent of all Americans do not consume enough water daily. Do you fit into this category?

If this is the case, you may experience constant fatigue, have more frequent headaches, and have less strength and endurance, making it difficult to establish and maintain any routine.

Carrying water with you at all times is one method to combat this all-too-common occurrence. Consume a full glass of water first thing in the morning, one after your morning exercise routine (which we will discuss shortly), and at every meal.

Continue sipping throughout the remainder of the day to reach the Mayo Clinic-recommended daily intake of 9 cups for women and 13 cups for men.

Tea's polyphenols are beneficial to the organism.

When you're not drinking water, you might want to consume tea. According to Harvard Medical School, the polyphenols present in tea have many beneficial effects on the body. Specifically, they possess anti-inflammatory and antioxidant properties.

Here are some of the finest teas to consume, along with the reasons why:

Relax, consume one or two cups per day, and obtain the benefits.

Get up from your seat...often
Being sedentary and confined to a desk all day can inflict havoc on your body.

The National Center on Health, Physical Activity, and Disability (NCHPAD) lists some of the physical effects of excessive seating, including an increased risk of colon and breast cancer, type 2 diabetes, strokes, and heart attacks, as well as mental decline and loss of muscle and bone.

In his article The Healthiest Way to Work, Kevan Lee, an expert content creator for Buffer, offers advice on how to get up and move more frequently. Consider incorporating techniques such as getting up every 20 minutes, using a standing desk, and sitting on a saddle or balance chair in your own life.

Exercise (MOVE!)
Exercise is the one component of a daily regimen that nearly everyone despises. And there are a multitude of reasons not to exercise:

"I dislike exercising."

"I was unable to wake up early enough, so I ran out of time. And I have no leisure in the evening."

"I really dislike sweating."
The list continues, but you get the idea.

In Choose Yourself, James Altucher describes excuses as "easy lies we tell ourselves to cover up our failures." How does one overcome these lies? Instead of focusing on what you dislike about exercise, you should focus on what it has to offer you.

Entrepreneur Joshua Steimle exercises because "if I stop exercising, my health will deteriorate." This decreases his productivity along with his motivation while simultaneously heightening his depressive feelings.

The ability to control your weight more easily, a decreased risk of type 2 diabetes and cancer, an enhanced mood, and more are additional advantages of regular exercise.

Exercise does not necessarily entail an hour-long, strenuous exercise session. Take a 10-20 minute walk. Perform yoga, stretching, or dance in your living room. Use the elliptical machine.

Alternatively, perform the Scientific 7-Minute Workout:

It does not matter what you do as long as you get your body moving!

Get adequate rest: a minimum of 7 hours There are numerous reasons why sleep is crucial to your overall health. In the short term, insufficient sleep can impair one's judgment, demeanor, and ability to retain information. Chronic sleep deprivation can result in obesity, diabetes, cardiovascular disease, and even premature mortality over time.

In addition to the physical and mental issues, it's difficult to maintain a full routine when all you can think about is crawling back into bed, drawing the covers over your head, and drifting off to sleep.

To get a decent night's sleep, you can:

Limit your caffeine intake to the morning hours.

Choose foods that induce sleep, such as bananas, oatmeal, and potatoes, later in the day.

Using earplugs or a white noise machine to eliminate nighttime outside pollution.

Darken your space

Avoid electronic devices one hour before slumber.

Remember that consistency and routine are crucial for developing sound sleep habits. According to Dr. Lawrence Epstein, co-author of The Harvard Medical School Guide to a Good Night's Sleep, "our body craves routine and likes to know what's coming."

Epstein identifies two simple tenets for healthy sleep: (1) having sufficient sleep (no less than seven hours) and (2) sleeping at the same time each day (as much as possible).

PART III: PERFECT YOUR SPIRIT

Emotional and spiritual self-care can elevate and propel you forward in the same way that mental and physical aspects of your daily routine can. Here are some alternatives to consider:

Get quiet: Try meditation
Okay, this is technically termed meditation, but if the concept of "meditation" is off-putting, just think of it as daily time spent in solitude. I used to believe that I would never be able to meditate (boy, was I incorrect!)

There are numerous advantages to engaging in this daily ritual. The Live and Dare blog's Giovanni lists 76 of them, including increased concentration, improved decision-making and problem-solving abilities, enhanced memory, and an easier time managing hyperactivity or attention deficit disorder. It achieves this by altering the structure of your brain. (It truly multiplies!)

According to Harvard University studies, meditation also reduces tension, anxiety, and depression, which are additional reasons to give it a try if you haven't already.

There are so many incredible guided meditations available online for free, and for many people, this is a wonderful way to get started (or improve your practice).

According to research, inspiration can be triggered, captured, and manipulated...It has a significant impact on significant life outcomes.

Daily, I peruse a few apps on my phone that inspire and motivate me. They keep me centered and grounded, thereby strengthening my mental foundation.

I repeat positive affirmations both in the morning and at night because I believe they are an effective means of fostering inspiration. In fact, Stanford University researchers have discovered that affirmations enhance education, health, and even relationships.

Find a word or phrase that you find empowering and motivating, and reiterate it to yourself repeatedly.

Practice gratitude by documenting what you're grateful for.
What would you have if you woke up tomorrow with only the items you were grateful for today?

By devoting time each day to expressing gratitude for all of your benefits, you accomplish two goals. First, you acknowledge that, although circumstances may not be ideal, you are fortunate to have what you do. Second, the more benefits for which you are grateful, the more you attract or draw in. As if they were multiplying.

In addition to recognizing your blessings, it is also beneficial to actively appreciate them. I ensure that I spend daily time with my daughter and wife, for instance, because I want them to know how appreciative I am to have them in my life.

I write a simple gratitude list every single day (even on the days I don't want to), and as a result of generating over a thousand of these lists, I have become a more optimistic, mindful, and observant individual.

Create a list of all the things for which you are grateful and review it when you wake up in the morning and before you go to bed at night. Additionally, you can select someone from your past for whom you are grateful, get in contact with them, and let them know. Consider the impact this could have on them... and on you!

Discover something new every day!
According to a study conducted by San Francisco State University, acquiring new knowledge increases long-term happiness. While it may cause you some anxiety in the short-term, at least until you attain a level of comfort, the end result is a greater level of life

satisfaction, which makes the initial discomfort more than worthwhile.

What are some topics you have not yet learned?

What about drawing, painting, or writing? Or perhaps you prefer something more physically demanding, such as rock climbing or acquiring a specific dance style. Or you could put your strength to the ultimate test by trying out for American Ninja Warrior. Why then?

Spend less time with those who bring you down.
The author James Altucher emphasizes the need to limit interactions with those who bring you down.

Consider the individuals in your life; do they provide you with emotional energy or deplete it? If the former is the case, spend more time with them. If the latter is true, maintaining your distance will make you happier.

Donate to others

There is something incredibly rewarding about assisting those around you. It is not necessary for the acts of service to be monumental. Something as basic as holding the door open for someone or offering a stranger (or loved one) a genuine compliment can have a profound effect on their day...and yours.

Make it a daily objective to do something kind for someone...And your grin will match theirs in magnitude.

You might also consider volunteering at a local charity or non-profit organization if you have the time. Websites such as VolunteerMatch, GiveBack, and AllForGood can help you locate the ideal volunteer opportunity.

Evaluate, monitor, and enhance.

Are you perusing this list with the following thought in mind?

"Well, I've tried many of these approaches, but I'm still not where I want to be."

If so, it may be time to take an honest look at your day-to-day activities and determine where your time is being spent. This is where technology can be of assistance.

There are numerous (this is an understatement) productivity-based applications available that can assist you in determining where you spend the majority of your time.

Exist, for example, has an app that helps you monitor your day and provides insight into how much time you spend being distracted versus productive. It also indicates the amount of time spent napping and engaging in physical activity. It even monitors your emotions.

I also use the Way of Life application to keep note of my daily habits. Invest approximately one minute per day to monitor, identify, and alter your habits...As you collect more and more data, you will be able to readily identify positive and negative lifestyle trends.

There are also websites that can assist you in becoming your finest self. Consider The Daily Practice as one option. This website enables you to set your own recurring objectives and assists you in turning them into habits. Alternatively, you can view theXeffect on reddit.

Three Questions to Consider
"Am I doing what I love?" is the first inquiry.
Let's be honest: it's difficult to be the finest version of yourself if you're unhappy with your life choices...

In his commencement address to Stanford students, the late Steve Jobs alluded to this concept as follows:

"...for the past two decades, I have asked myself each morning, 'If today were the last day of my existence, would I want to do what I am about to do today?' And whenever the answer is "No" for too many consecutive days, I know I need to make a change."

So, are you engaged in activities that you would be pleased with if it were your last day on earth?

If not, you should consider what you could be doing that would make you feel more fulfilled and full of life. Create an inventory of activities that will make you happy and incorporate them into your schedule so that your answer to this question is an emphatic "YES!"

What is the worst that could possibly happen?

Have you ever awakened in the small hours of the morning anxious about something that may occur later that day, week, month, or year? Or perhaps you spend a great deal of time throughout the day ruminating on future events with an overwhelming sense of dread as you consider everything that could possibly go awry.

Find a comfortable place to rest or lie down and concentrate on listening. Attention generates energy, and when energy is in motion, it can naturally transmute. Whoever wishes to lose weight only needs to understand that energy always transforms and that, under certain conditions, it may stagnate or flow less.

This meditation reintroduces one to the original source of all energy, within the heart, where a personality of eternity, wisdom, and joy emanates this wonderful energy that constitutes all universes and the human form of life.

By awakening the dormant intelligence of the original nature within nature, one may be able to exert control over the senses and all aspects of existence.

The tongue is the most powerful sense because it constantly desires and yearns for more. More conversation, sustenance, and labor; more, more, more.

This results in a vicious cycle of gorging, overexertion, and eventual exhaustion. One can now learn to use the tongue properly by controlling the tongue's strong urges and becoming aware of one's true nature, which is to be eternally joyful.

First, we become conscious of the respiration and learn to use it as the ideal fuel. We inhale profoundly through the nose in order to absorb the energy. Here, at a tranquil source, we allow the natural passage of the breath to the heart as we sit with our backs against the wall. One can close their eyes and envision a sacred space of peace and beauty, surrounded by nature and safeguarded by holiness.

The source is named Ananda, and we become acquainted with Ananda. How does one get to know another person? One must inquire and listen with sincerity. Ananda introduces Himself as follows: "I am the source of all material and spiritual energy; even knowledge, memory, and forgetfulness emanate from Me; I am seated joyfully in the hearts of all beings."

Ananda is spiritual, so perpetually euphoric and joyful. Ananda is seated on a magnificent throne of Jewels while garlands of fragrant flowers adorn his neck. Beyond this sacred site, one can hear the sound of water ecstatically bursting into existence, and here, all opulence, beauty, energy, and wisdom burst forth into the living being's body. Ananda gives us a flower from his floral garland, and we can see a special glow emanating from it and smell its sweet aroma.

It is a transcendental flower that grows ceaselessly in the center of joy. The garden of hope and happiness resides within each individual's heart, where the personification of happiness sits on a jeweled throne with all opulences, energy, beauty, and wisdom. This spiritual being, Ananda, resides eternally within each individual's consciousness. Ananda is also seated within the souls of animals and other humans as a blissful companion who guides the journeys of all living things.

Let's take a stroll to view this garden of hearts' joy and faith. Here, all desires are fulfilled; one need only inquire earnestly. "Dearest heart of all, Ananda, please grant me the body I desire. Let me be extremely beautiful and strong, with ample vitality to spare for everyone."

Ananda is extremely merciful and grants all spiritual fulfillment desires. To be healthy, fit, and thriving green in the natural paradise of the spiritual garden of the heart, which is full of hope and joy, one must simply adhere to certain principles during this lifetime.

So, let's take a hike in the highlands to gain an understanding of one's behavior outside of social and economic norms.

Make this a breath-by-breath walk of consciousness.

Every step increases one's awareness and attentiveness. One can sense his or her feet, ankle-area muscles, thighs, and hips. One is aware of a healthy tension in the lower body, similar to how horses are worked and trained to be reliable conveyances for the embodied spark of joy.

Each stride is taken consciously, and each step is accompanied by a breath. Inhaling and exhaling generously and consciously. The inhale and exhale are equivalent. There is a peaceful interval in between. Inhale, euphoric pause, then exhale. Blissful halt. Inhale, feel the light, exhale, and be conscious.

Allow the incoming energy to transform, then return it to nature and unwind. Inhale for energy, allow it to transmute, release stagnation, and exhale to feel the body. The respiration can be shallow or very deep within the abdomen. This is the skill of cognizant breathing, which can be learned. Just imagine, step-by-step, climbing this mountain of your wish and seeing yourself at the summit of your experience.

On this path, one will experience a variety of emotions; therefore, a stable reference point is required. A focal point. Concentrate on the heart and the tip of the nose, the exact locations where air enters and exits the body. Observe the inhalation and exhalation at the nostrils, from which the air passes naturally to the heart and into the body. Fresh vitality and buoyancy.

All mountaineers will attest to the fact that respiration alone provides energy. Let's ascend this mountain of accomplishment to reach the desired result. What are these? Perhaps flawless health and a high quality of life devoid of worries. Possibly a method to experience happiness and joy every day. One may declare, "I can do it!"

The mountain represents the current embodiment, and by overcoming the mountain of oneself, one becomes qualified to serve humanity in the most effective manner. This is of interest to me and you. Moreover, one can reach one's full potential by employing the body, mind, and spirit in service to all.

We are nearing the summit and are only a few breaths away.

Inhale, feel light, exhale, and surrender.
Inhale, feel light, exhale, and surrender.
Inhale, feel light, exhale, and surrender.

From the mountain's peak, we can see distant nature that is gorgeous, tranquil, and at peace. What have we neglected? Where are one's interior tranquility and peace?

This summit instills confidence and a sense of self. One can be steady regardless of the shifts in nature if he or she is as dependable and resilient as a mountain. The seasons change, but a wise individual is not perturbed. The winds arrive and go, but one breathes in gently the air of equilibrium and equanimity.

Simply view the world through the lens of your inner heart and be conscious of your inner yearning to live a life of fulfillment and contentment. Imagine yourself in this position, content and successful. Simply observe the current of your respiration and how it feels. Smile as you see yourself in your inner vision and continue to breathe. Consider the embodiment of bliss, Ananda, who is seated in a garden of tranquil ecstasy and abundance as you gaze into your own heart. Hope is personified within each individual's spirit, and it is a sublime perception to recognize this.

The true nature is personal and distinctive, but it manifests itself in every aspect of creation, in every living being and entity. Everything has a distinct and enthusiastic personality, form, character, and propensity to love.

Realizing "I am a part of the whole, absolute truth" is sufficient to induce happiness.

Knowing this, one may already be satisfied, just as all plants and animals are satisfied by the impending autumn rain; everyone receives a portion. The rain evenly and abundantly distributes water everywhere. The plants are nourished simply by absorbing rainfall and air and light currents.

Self-satisfaction can be achieved by embracing one's true nature, which is eternal, wise, and blissful. It is a challenge we all face to live it out. This mountain peak presented a challenge, but in your vision you have already conquered your own magnificence. How do individuals ascend the world's tallest mountains? They have a distinct mental image of the result and outcome; how success appears in their minds may also manifest physically.

Manifestation works from subtle to coarse, so it must first take place in consciousness, intelligence, and mind before the senses and body execute the inner conscious will. Through gentle, balanced, and precise breathing, one can gain access to the spiritual regions of consciousness in which anything is possible. This is said of Ananda because the personification of eternity, wisdom, and bliss is a genuine bestower of blessings for any desire, such as success, weight loss, happy relationships, excellent grades, etc.

Ananda is the source of conscious effort, and the personality is in charge of the intelligence, intellect, and senses. One can envision the blissful Self, Ananda, seated within a carriage. This tranquil and tranquil personality is drawn by a carriage whose reins are tightly held by intelligence. The mind strings and directs the senses, which are like horses hauling a carriage.

This image is an analogy from the Gitopanishad and resembles the following hierarchy.

"The working senses are superior to dull matter; the mind is superior to the senses; intelligence is superior to the mind; and Ananda is superior to intelligence."

Therefore, to accomplish something, one must directly address Ananda. This is why we meditate and pray for the connection to Ananda, the ecstatic equilibrium and individuality that resides within the heart.

Find this blissful equilibrium and simply hearken to this wonderful tale of King Ambarisa, an ardent devotee of Ananda. Ambarisa, as king, resided in a magnificent mountaintop castle in a land where all beings were treated equally due to a shared comprehension of their equality.

Even dogs and livestock were protected and cared for, as all life was regarded as sacred, both in the spiritual sky and on earth. Spiritually, there is no distinction between a cat, a cow, a child, an adult, or even a saintly monarch like Ambarisa because they are all conscious, Ananda-filled beings.

As the sheaths form around Ananda, the blissful center of eternity and knowledge, a single living entity may assume the form of a cow, a cat, or an infant. The virtuous King Ambarisa was aware of this, and as a result, he executed his duty as a ruler with great care by treating everyone equally.

The younger generation held a special place in his heart, and he could not go a moment without considering how to please Ananda in the souls of all. Consequently, he prepared a feast for Ananda, the Supreme Personification of ecstasy and eternity. All the citizens of the kingdom were invited to feast, dance, and chant lavishly, with the knowledge that his labor force might need a couple of days off. Ambarisa took feeding everyone very seriously.

A king as generous as Ambarisa also made sacrifices to satisfy Ananda. He removed his sandals and embarked on a cross-country trek to reach holy pilgrimage sites, seeking the blessings of priests and monks in the monasteries. By presenting everything generously to the Whole, Ambarisa could serve as a model for how to achieve life's perfection. Ambarisa was able to win over everyone's affections by sacrificing appropriately. His entire body was devoted to the service of Ananda, pleasure, and he carried out numerous saints' and monks' directives. To purify his voice, he performed prayers and beautiful chants in the temples, washed his feet with holy water, offered flowers and fruits on the altar and in the communal kitchen, and listened to the wise saints and the elderly. His hands were engaged in cleaning the temple and accepting sacramental food, while his tongue sampled this sacramental food. His eyes were fixed on the deity Ananda, and he devoted his entire existence to exemplary service.

His glories resided in the hidden core of altruism and compassion for all living things.

Simply breathe and be content while contemplating the alluring personality within the heart. Here, Ananda sits like a monarch on a throne covered in jewels and lavishly adorned with flower garlands. Beside him is his close friend Ambarisa, who serves him.

While listening to this narrative, one might wonder how it can help them lose weight and feel more at ease.

Relax and enable us to find a solution that allows for additional meditation and reflection.

There is providence, divine care for all beings, which naturally gives each being a unique position and form.

Yaks were created in the mountains to assist the herders in carrying their loads through the mountain paths. This remains the primary mode of conveyance in certain regions of the world's tallest mountains. Yaks are still employed for producing valuable milk and transporting cargo along steep mountain paths.

A person born into a priestly or scholarly family is likely to become a cleric or scholar. Someone born into a royal family may become a monarch or queen, while someone born into a cowherding family will likely remain a cowherd. Similarly, one receives a body that safeguards inner pleasure, Ananda, and thus the body is anticipated to serve as a vehicle for an entire lifetime.

One must be grateful and appreciative for what they have received from providence, but they can alter their lifestyle by getting in shape. To be able to raise a good human existence, one must maintain a healthy body. The purpose of a person's existence should be self-actualization; accordingly, one must eat, sleep, and work.

The majority of people in today's society consume to live, and consequently, they die at a very young age. We should rather strive to realize the full potential of each individual. This is known as consciousness.

Consciousness travels with the breath; therefore, let's continue to hone the distinct breathing capacity of healing consciousness.

I am Light, blissful, and healthy as I inhale.
Exhaling, I am giving generously...

I am Light, blissful, and healthy as I inhale.
As I exhale, I am protected and tended for...

I am Light, blissful, and healthy as I inhale.
As I exhale, I am aware of letting go...

I am Light, blissful, and healthy as I inhale.
By exhaling, I create space for perfection.

By reciting a sacrosanct sound formula, one can progressively become lighter. Yes, chanting helps develop self-awareness, trust, and a lighthearted disposition.

Chanting is conscious chanting performed in the devotional spirit of adoration for the Supreme Whole or Ananda. This is technically known as a mantra and is considered the most effective method to simultaneously be happy, conscious, and healthy.

Chanting induces levity and pure body awareness. The voice is distinctive because it permeates all layers of being and can be used deliberately. Have you ever been moved by music? This profound transformation of consciousness occurs within the center of balance and harmony, the heart.

A simple chant affirming lightness is the ideal companion for lengthy walks, whether solitary or in a group.

Simply recite the following:

I am the World's Source of Light
I am the World's Light, I am the World's Light, I am the World's Light.

You are the World's Light, You are the World's Light, You are the World's Light, You are the World's Light.

We are the World's Light, We are the World's Light, We are the World's Light, We are the World's Light.

May lightness surround you, and may it frequently accompany you throughout your existence.

Practice and recite this mantra using your own voice. There are no hard and fast rules for chanting, and it is said that reciting this mantra calms a flitting mind and fosters self-love and trust. The mantra (literally, "a technique to still the mind") will be repeated and used as a point of reference throughout this book.

The constant repetition serves as an anchor along the path of self-love, trust, and shedding the burden of material existence.

Weight loss entails shedding the burden of material nature. Due to its ephemeral nature, nature comes and goes, appears and disappears, in dualities such as heat and cold, summer and winter, and up and down. We are all a part of this material world, and we all suffer as a result of our conditioning.

The only effective remedy, which explains the Light metaphor, is to identify with eternal nature.

There is both a temporal world and an eternal, wise, and blissfully enlightened spiritual world. When one identifies with this eternal nature, the burdens of the transient material world vanish and enlightenment occurs.

Tips For Tantric Sexual Practice: Masturbation And Partner Play

What does Tantric mean?

Although it is frequently equated with Tantric intercourse, it is really about the relationship - whether it is between you and your partner or between you and yourself.

In fact, the word itself, which is derived from an ancient Sanskrit word, denotes an energy net or trap. Tantra Gyan is the practice of transcending the sexual and spiritual realms through natural, meditative intercourse.

As Tantric Yoga is concerned with both physical and spiritual awareness, so is this concept concerned with knowing one's body. When you study and practice Tantra, you become one with your body, which brings you contentment and is a means of experiencing happiness.

This enables you to pay closer attention to the needs and desires of your body and ensure they are met. Moreover, the energy that you channel during Tantric intercourse flows through your body and can accelerate your orgasms. And if you have a partner, you are familiar with his or her anatomy.

Tantra is not solely concerned with increasing levels of body-mind awareness.

It may also involve fostering a more intimate and harmonious relationship with your partner. During Tantra practice, you and your companion learn to be physically aware and spiritually present by energizing each other, a process that continues long after sexual activity.

This system also enables you to explore and communicate aspects of your personalities, allowing you to become intimately acquainted.

Your spouse is interested in implementing this technique, but you are unsure how to tell them. On her blog, author and sexual empowerment coach

Sofia Sundari provides the following advice.

Avoid overwhelming your companion. Instead, describe your sexual preferences and how to enhance the experience. Listen to what they are saying. Your partner may enthusiastically answer either yes or no. Or they could be somewhere else.

Regardless of their response, respect and listen to them. Allow the instructor to assume charge. If your partner is compatible with the system, locate a fitness instructor who can teach you both about exercise.

How to Get Your Mind Ready

Tantra is a spiritual exercise in which the intellect functions similarly to the body. When you master this technique, your body, mind, and spirit are united.

Unifying these elements requires a clear mind and a willingness to venture outside your comfort zone. Some people believe that meditating for 10 to 15 minutes helps prepare the brain for tantra practice because it provides the opportunity to evaluate it internally.

Test it out. Observe your respiration. Take 15 to 30 minutes to breathe light into your belly and lower back and remain in touch with what's happening in your brain, whether it's stress or cravings.

Stretch for some time.
As you stretch each limb, rid your mind of any burdensome negative notions. The more times the pack is opened, the simpler it is to swap. Every day, devote at least 30 minutes to journalism. Make an effort to record notions that inhibit your spiritual development.

How to construct your own space system is a detailed exercise.
Sexual activity is not always prohibited - in any case. Your environment has a direct bearing on your state of mind and capacity to unwind and appreciate this voyage.

Do this where the temperature is suitable. If the climate is cool, you should exercise for an hour prior to heating your bed. If it is hot, turn on the air conditioning but set the temperature above 70 degrees so that the room is chilly, not frigid.

Candles or light sources can be used to illuminate the perimeter of a room. Soft red LEDs add a subtle touch to the floor while adding romance to the room. Fill the empty space with a delightful aroma. The light of a candle illuminates fragrant incense, which diffuses light to illuminate hanging blossoms. Choose a scent that will make you seductive without surprising others. Your space regularly. Remove the satin drape and insert some pillows. Create a romantic environment. Play any music that you and your companion can enjoy together.

How to Pass the Time When Alone
There are numerous methods to acquire tantric principles when alone. Bear in

mind, however, that masturbation is not always the final game; you can play it alone, work it out, or go either way. Meditation is the most effective method for eliminating all obstacles.

However, instead of depleting your vitality, you gain it. As you ponder, your energy flows downward into the earth. This energy permeates your entire body and grants you vitality.

Try getting a full-body massage.
Apply your preferred moisturizer or oil to your epidermis. For instance, oil massages or time spent with bumps on the eyes, back, thighs, limbs, neck, and chest.

Not all single-player games involve climax.
Instead, take the time to investigate what makes your genitalia content. Explore yourself in novel methods. Reduce the firing rate. Don't neglect to take deep breaths and move slowly while playing.

You can breathe and feel it throughout your body while meditating or masturbating. Don't let your mind wander; instead, pay attention to your entire body and allow it to experience emotions.

This will enable you to maximize your strength and energy. Determine what you hope to accomplish in your tantra class, such as having improved orgasms or feeling more at ease in your own skin. I would never go there. You and your companion can apply tantric principles to other moment-generating practices.

Regardless, you and your partner must be entirely present and seated in front of one another.

Eye contact.

As you breathe, begin slowly moving your body, and after five minutes, alternately massage your arms, legs, neck, etc., and begin consciously handling your body.

Start Kissing Kiss after five minutes. Concentrate on every physical sensation you feel at this time.

Sexual activity (optional)
You can enhance intimacy, or! Strategy is primarily concerned with communication. If you choose to delay sexual activity.

And do not fear being creative. Try novel locations.
Explore unexplored desires by touching each other with fresh palms. Most importantly, immerse yourself in the stress-free experience of spending time before transitioning to the next emotional exercise. Alternatively, you can exchange energy by hugging your companion.
Develop a profound bond that can be woven.
Consider the position of the utensil to accomplish this. The companion in the rear transmits energy (donor), while the partner in front absorbs it (receiver).

Align yourself with your intestines and heart.

The giver should rest his hand on the recipient's heart after wrapping his hand around him. The recipient must extend his hand.

Calm yourself for a moment, then coordinate your breathing and allow energy to freely circulate between you.

www.ingramcontent.com/pod-product-compliance
Lightning Source LLC
Chambersburg PA
CBHW060505030426
42337CB00015B/1743